Treatment Methods for Kidney Failure
TRANSPLANTATION

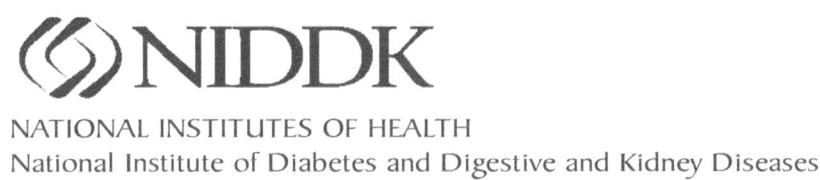

NATIONAL INSTITUTES OF HEALTH
National Institute of Diabetes and Digestive and Kidney Diseases

Contents

If you have advanced and permanent kidney failure, kidney transplantation may be the treatment option that allows you to live much like you lived before your kidneys failed. Since the 1950s, when the first kidney transplants were performed, much has been learned about how to prevent rejection and minimize the side effects of medicines.

But transplantation is not a cure; it's an ongoing treatment that requires you to take medicines for the rest of your life. And the wait for a donated kidney can be years long.

A successful transplant takes a coordinated effort from your whole health care team, including your nephrologist, transplant surgeon, transplant coordinator, pharmacist, dietitian, and social worker. But the most important members of your health care team are you and your family. By learning about your treatment, you can work with your health care team to give yourself the best possible results, and you can lead a full, active life.

When Your Kidneys Fail

Healthy kidneys clean your blood by removing excess fluid, minerals, and wastes. They also make hormones that keep your bones strong and your blood healthy. When your kidneys fail, harmful wastes build up in your body, your blood pressure may rise, and your body may retain excess fluid and not make enough red blood cells. When this happens, you need treatment to replace the work of your failed kidneys.

How Transplantation Works

Kidney transplantation is a procedure that places a healthy kidney from another person into your body. This one new kidney takes over the work of your two failed kidneys.

A surgeon places the new kidney inside your lower abdomen and connects the artery and vein of the new kidney to your artery and vein. Your blood flows through the new kidney, which makes urine, just like your own kidneys did when they were healthy. Unless they are causing infection or high blood pressure, your own kidneys are left in place.

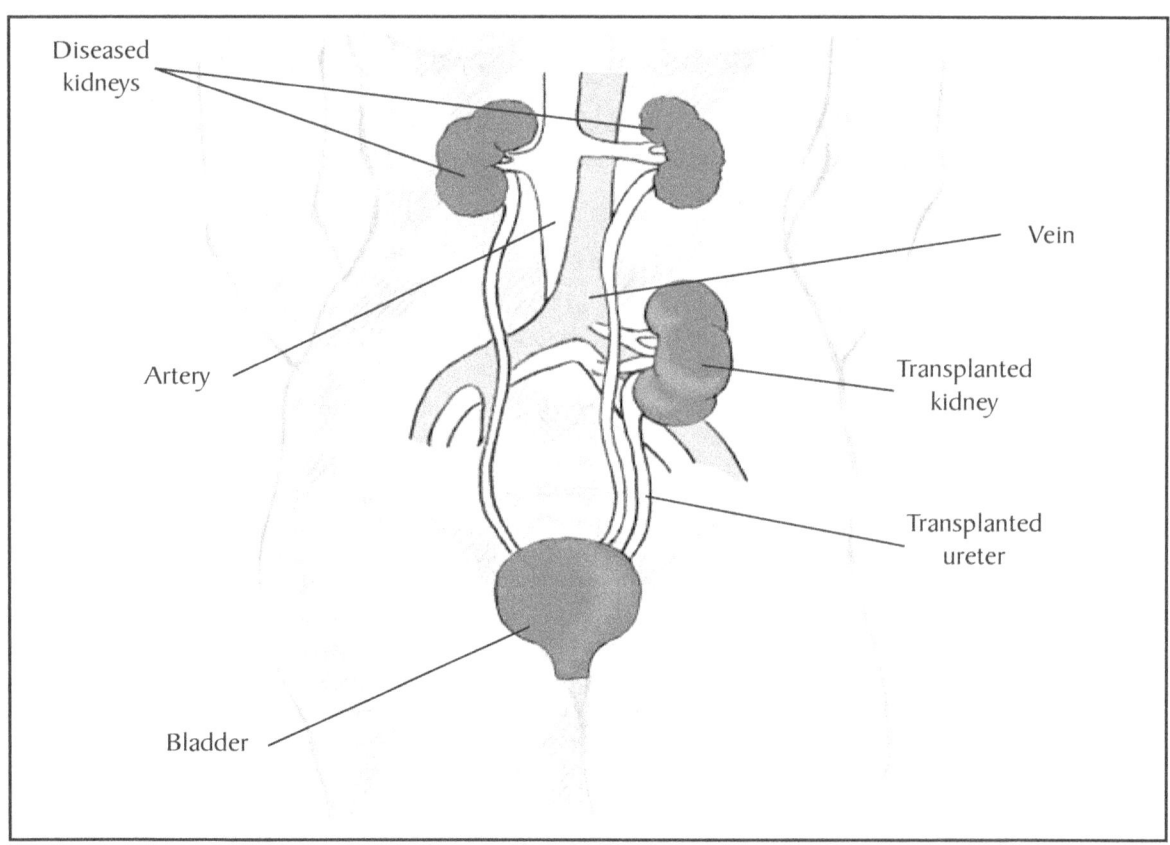

Diseased kidneys

Vein

Artery

Transplanted kidney

Transplanted ureter

Bladder

Kidney transplantation.

The Transplant Process

Your Doctor's Recommendation

The transplantation process begins when you learn that your kidneys are failing and you must start to consider your treatment options. Whether transplantation is to be among your options will depend on your specific situation. Transplantation isn't for everyone. Your doctor may tell you that you have a condition that would make transplantation dangerous or unlikely to succeed.

Medical Evaluation at a Transplant Center

If your doctor sees transplantation as an option, the next step is a thorough medical evaluation at a transplant hospital. The pretransplant evaluation may require several visits over the course of several weeks or even months. You'll need to have blood drawn and x rays taken. You'll be tested for blood type and other matching factors that determine whether your body will accept an available kidney.

The medical team will want to see whether you're healthy enough for surgery. Cancer, a serious infection, or significant cardiovascular disease would make transplantation unlikely to succeed. In addition, the medical team will want to make sure that you can understand and follow the schedule for taking medicines.

If a family member or friend wants to donate a kidney, he or she will need to be evaluated for general health and to see whether the kidney is a good match. (See the "Organ Donation" section on page 9.)

Placement on the Waiting List

If the medical evaluation shows that you're a good candidate for a transplant but you don't have a family member or friend who can donate a kidney, you'll be put on the transplant program's waiting list to receive a kidney from a deceased donor—someone who has just died.

Every person waiting for a deceased donor organ is registered with the Organ Procurement and Transplantation Network (OPTN), which maintains a centralized computer network linking all regional organ gathering organizations (known as organ procurement organizations, or OPOs) and transplant centers. The United Network for Organ Sharing (UNOS), a private nonprofit organization, administers OPTN under a contract with the Federal Government. (See the "Resources" section at the back of this booklet on page 14.)

UNOS rules allow patients to register with multiple transplant centers. Each transplant center will probably require a separate medical evaluation, even if a patient is already registered at another center.

Observers of OPTN operations have raised the concern that people in certain regions of the country have to wait longer than others because allocation policies for some organs give preference to patients within the donor's region. Kidneys, however, are assigned to the best match regardless of geographic region. The Federal Government continues to monitor policies and regulations to ensure that every person waiting for an organ has a fair chance. The key to making waiting times shorter is to increase the number of donated organs.

Waiting Period

How long you'll have to wait depends on many things but is primarily determined by the degree of matching between you and the donor. Some people wait several years for a good match, while others get matched within a few months.

While you're on the waiting list, notify the transplant center of changes in your health. Also, let the transplant center know if you move or change telephone numbers. The center will need to find you immediately when a kidney becomes available.

OPOs are responsible for identifying potential organs for transplant and coordinating with the national network. The 69 regional OPOs are all UNOS members. When a deceased donor kidney becomes available, the OPO notifies UNOS, and a computer-generated list of suitable recipients is created. Suitability is initially based on two factors:

- **Blood type.** Your blood type (A, B, AB, or O) must be compatible with the donor's blood type.

- **HLA factors.** HLA stands for human leukocyte antigen, a genetic marker located on the surface of your white blood cells. You inherit a set of three antigens from your mother and three from your father. A higher number of matching antigens increases the chance that your kidney will last for a long time.

If you're selected on the basis of the first two factors, a third is evaluated:

- **Antibodies.** Your immune system may produce antibodies that act specifically against something in the donor's tissues. To see whether this is the case, a small sample of your blood will be mixed with a small sample of the donor's blood in a tube. If no reaction occurs, you should be able to accept the kidney. Your transplant team might use the term negative cross-match to describe this lack of reaction.

Transplant Operation

If you have a living donor, you'll schedule the operation in advance. You and your donor will be operated on at the same time, usually in side-by-side rooms. One team of surgeons will perform the nephrectomy—that is, the removal of the kidney from the donor—while another prepares the recipient for placement of the donated kidney.

If you're on a waiting list for a deceased donor kidney, you must be ready to hurry to the hospital as soon as a kidney becomes available. Once there, you'll give a blood sample for the antibody cross-match test. If you have a negative cross-match, it means that your antibodies don't react and the transplantation can proceed.

You'll be given a general anesthetic to make you sleep during the operation, which usually takes 3 or 4 hours. The surgeon will make a small cut in your lower abdomen. The artery and vein from the new kidney will be attached to your artery and vein. The ureter from the new kidney will be connected to your bladder.

Often, the new kidney will start making urine as soon as your blood starts flowing through it, but sometimes a few weeks pass before it starts working.

Recovery From Surgery

As after any major surgery, you'll probably feel sore and groggy when you wake up. However, many transplant recipients report feeling much better immediately after surgery. Even if you wake up feeling great, you'll need to stay in the hospital for about a week to recover from surgery, and longer if you have any complications.

Posttransplant Care

Your body's immune system is designed to keep you healthy by sensing "foreign invaders," such as bacteria, and rejecting them. But your immune system will also sense that your new kidney is foreign. To keep your body from rejecting it, you'll have to take drugs that turn off, or suppress, your immune response. You may have to take two or more of these immunosuppressant medicines, as well as medications to treat other health problems. Your health care team will help you learn what each pill is for and when to take it. Be sure that you understand the instructions for taking your medicines before you leave the hospital.

If you've been on hemodialysis, you'll find that your posttransplant diet is much less restrictive. You can drink more fluids and eat many of the fruits and vegetables you were previously told to avoid. You may even need to gain a little weight, but be careful not to gain weight too quickly and avoid salty foods that can lead to high blood pressure.

Work with your clinic's dietitian to make sure you're following a healthy eating plan.

Rejection

You can help prevent rejection by taking your medicines and following your diet, but watching for signs of rejection—like fever or soreness in the area of the new kidney or a change in the amount of urine you make—is important. Report any such changes to your health care team.

Even if you do everything you're supposed to do, your body may still reject the new kidney and you may need to go back on dialysis. Unless your health care team determines that you're no longer a good candidate for transplantation, you can go back on the waiting list for another kidney.

Side Effects of Immunosuppressants

Immunosuppressants can weaken your immune system, which can lead to infections. Some drugs may also change your appearance. Your face may get fuller; you may gain weight or develop acne or facial hair. Not all patients have these problems, though, and diet and makeup can help.

Immunosuppressants work by diminishing the ability of immune cells to function. In some patients, over long periods of time, this diminished immunity can increase the risk of developing cancer. Some immunosuppressants cause cataracts, diabetes, extra stomach acid, high blood pressure, and bone disease. When used over time, these drugs may also cause liver or kidney damage in a few patients.

Financial Issues

Treatment for kidney failure is expensive, but Federal health insurance plans pay much of the cost, usually up to 80 percent. Often, private insurance or state programs pay the rest. Your social worker can help you locate resources for financial assistance. For more information, see the National Institute of Diabetes and Digestive and Kidney Diseases (NIDDK) fact sheet *Financial Help for Treatment of Kidney Failure*.

Additional Patient Assistance Programs

UNOS maintains a website called Transplant Living to help patients learn about their treatment and find resources. The website includes a page that lists organizations that provide financial assistance—available at *www.transplantliving.org/beforethetransplant/finance/funding.aspx*.

Organ Donation

Deceased Donor

Most transplanted kidneys come from people who have died. However, the number of people waiting for kidneys has increased in recent years, while the number of kidneys available from deceased donors has remained constant. The result is a shortage of kidneys and a longer waiting time for people with kidney failure.

Many suitable kidneys go unused because family members of potential donors don't know their loved one's wishes. People who wish to donate their organs should talk about this issue with their families. Several organizations, including UNOS

Patient Assistance Programs
———— From Prescription Drug Companies ————

The immunosuppressants and other drugs you must take after your transplant will be a large part of your medical expenses. Most drug manufacturers have patient assistance programs giving discounts to patients who can show that they can't afford the cost of their prescribed medications. The Pharmaceutical Research and Manufacturers of America publishes the *Directory of Prescription Drug Patient Assistance Programs,* available at *www.pparx.org.* To request a directory through the mail, write to

Pharmaceutical Research and Manufacturers of America
1100 Fifteenth Street NW
Washington, DC 20005

An organization called the Medicine Program offers help in finding and applying for free medicines supplied by pharmaceutical companies. To request assistance, obtain an application form, available on the website or through the mail, and list the medicines you need. Send the application back with a $5 processing fee for each medicine you request. If the Medicine Program fails to qualify you to receive the medicine, your processing fee will be returned.

The Medicine Program
P.O. Box 1089
Poplar Bluff, MO 63902
Phone: 1–866–694–3893
Internet: www.themedicineprogram.com

and the National Kidney Foundation (see the "Resources" section on page 14), provide organ donor cards for people who wish to make this life-preserving gift when they die. A properly completed organ donor card notifies medical officials that you've decided to donate your organs. In most states, you can indicate your desire to be an organ donor on your driver's license.

Living Donor

A growing number of transplanted kidneys are donated by living family members or friends. Potential donors need to be tested to make sure that donating a kidney won't endanger their health, as well as for matching factors. Most people, however, can donate a kidney with little risk.

A kidney from a living donor often has advantages over a deceased donor kidney:

- People who receive a kidney from a family member or friend don't have to wait until a kidney becomes available. Living donation allows for greater preparation and for the operation to be scheduled at a convenient time.

- Kidneys from family members are more likely to be good matchcs, although there's no guarantee.

- Kidneys from living donors don't need to be transported from one site to another, so the kidney is in better condition when it's transplanted.

- Living donation helps people waiting for kidneys from deceased donors by lowering the number of people on the waiting list.

Minority Donation

Diseases of the kidney are found more frequently in racial and ethnic minority populations in the United States than in the general population. African Americans, Asian Americans, Hispanics/Latinos, and Pacific Islander Americans are three times more likely to suffer from kidney failure than Americans of European descent. Successful transplantation is often enhanced if organs are matched between members of the same ethnic and racial group. A shortage of organs donated by minorities can contribute to longer waiting periods for transplants for minorities.

The National Minority Organ/Tissue Transplant Education Program (MOTTEP), with the support of the National Institutes of Health's (NIH's) Office of Research on Minority Health and the NIDDK, is the first national program to empower minority communities to promote minority donation and transplantation, as well as good health habits. In turn, this effort should improve the chances for a well-matched organ among all those waiting for a transplant.

Hope Through Research

The NIDDK, through its Division of Kidney, Urologic, and Hematologic Diseases, supports several programs and studies devoted to improving treatment for patients with progressive kidney disease and permanent kidney failure, including patients who receive a transplanted kidney.

- **The End-Stage Renal Disease Program** promotes research to reduce medical problems from bone, blood, nervous system, metabolic, gastrointestinal, cardiovascular, and endocrine abnormalities in kidney failure and to improve the effectiveness of dialysis and transplantation. The program seeks to increase kidney graft and patient survival and to maximize quality of life.

- **The NIH Organ/Tissue Transplant Center,** located at the NIH Clinical Center in Bethesda, MD, is a collaborative project of NIH, the Walter Reed Army Medical Center, the Naval Medical Research Center, and the Diabetes Research Institute at the University of Miami. The site includes a state-of-the-art clinical transplant ward, operating facility, and outpatient clinic designed for the study of new drugs or techniques that may improve the success of organ and tissue transplants.

- **The U.S. Renal Data System (USRDS)** collects, analyzes, and distributes information about the use of dialysis and transplantation to treat kidney failure in the United States. The USRDS is funded directly by NIDDK in conjunction with the Centers for Medicare & Medicaid Services. The USRDS publishes an *Annual Data Report*, which characterizes the total population of people being treated for kidney failure; reports on incidence, prevalence, mortality rates, and trends over time; and develops data on the effects of various treatment modalities. The report also helps identify problems and opportunities for more focused special studies of renal research issues.

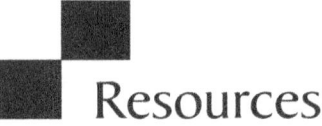

Resources

Government Agencies

A number of Federal agencies are involved in various aspects of transplantation, including financing, procurement regulation and oversight, allocation policy development, donation promotion, and biomedical research.

The Centers for Medicare & Medicaid Services runs the Medicare and Medicaid programs. You can apply for Medicare through your local Social Security office. The national phone number for the Social Security Administration is 1–800–772–1213, and you can get additional information about Medicare health plans by calling 1–800–633–4227 (1–800–MEDICARE). The official U.S. Government website for Medicare information can be found at *www.medicare.gov*.

The U.S. Department of Health and Human Services coordinates organ procurement and allocation activities through its Health Resources and Services Administration (HRSA).

Health Resources and Services Administration
Division of Transplantation
Room 12C–06, Parklawn Building
5600 Fishers Lane
Rockville, MD 20857
Phone: 301–443–7577
Internet: www.hrsa.gov

HRSA also maintains a website devoted to organ donation at *www.organdonor.gov*.

HRSA's Division of Transplantation administers the OPTN through a contract with UNOS, whose website can be found at *www.transplantliving.org*. You can request a packet of information about kidney transplantation by calling UNOS at 1–888–894–6361 (1–888–TX–INFO–1).

Nongovernment Organizations

Many national organizations—including Government agencies, private foundations, and commercial industries—have joined the Coalition on Donation to promote organ and tissue donation through educational programs and campaigns conducted nationally and at the local level.

Coalition on Donation
700 North 4th Street
Richmond, VA 23219
Phone: 804–782–4920
Fax: 804–782–4643
Internet: www.shareyourlife.org

TransWeb: All About Transplantation and Donation is a nonprofit educational website (*www.transweb.org*) featuring answers to frequently asked questions, donor memorials, patient experiences, and a reference section.

Additional Organizations That Can Help

American Association of Kidney Patients
3505 East Frontage Road
Suite 315
Tampa, FL 33607
Phone: 1–800–749–2257
Fax: 813–636–8122
Email: info@aakp.org
Internet: www.aakp.org

American Diabetes Association
ATTN: National Call Center
1701 North Beauregard Street
Alexandria, VA 22311
Phone: 1–800–342–2383
Email: askADA@diabetes.org
Internet: www.diabetes.org

American Kidney Fund
6110 Executive Boulevard
Suite 1010
Rockville, MD 20852
Phone: 1–800–638–8299
Email: helpline@akfinc.org
Internet: www.kidneyfund.org

American Society of Transplantation
15000 Commerce Parkway
Suite C
Mount Laurel, NJ 08054
Phone: 856–439–9986
Fax: 856–439–9982
Email: ast@ahint.com
Internet: www.a-s-t.org

Life Options Rehabilitation Program
c/o Medical Education Institute Inc.
414 D'Onofrio Drive
Suite 200
Madison, WI 53719
Phone: 1–800–468–7777
Fax: 608–833–8366
Email: lifeoptions@MEIresearch.org
Internet: www.lifeoptions.org
          www.kidneyschool.org

National Kidney Foundation Inc.
30 East 33rd Street
New York, NY 10016
Phone: 1–800–622–9010
Fax: 212–689–9261
Email: info@kidney.org
Internet: www.kidney.org

Additional Reading

If you would like to learn more about kidney failure and its treatment, you may be interested in reading

AAKP Patient Plan
This is a series of booklets and newsletters that cover the different phases of learning about kidney failure, choosing a treatment, and adjusting to changes.
American Association of Kidney Patients
3505 East Frontage Road
Suite 315
Tampa, FL 33607
Phone: 1–800–749–2257
Fax: 813–636–8122
Email: info@aakp.org
Internet: www.aakp.org

Getting a New Kidney: Facts About Kidney Transplants
and
Keeping Your New Kidney Healthy: Facts About Transplant Medications
American Society of Transplantation
15000 Commerce Parkway
Suite C
Mount Laurel, NJ 08054
Phone: 856–439–9986
Email: ast@ahint.com
Internet: www.a-s-t.org/patient_education/english/
    available_brochures.htm

Kidney Transplantation
American Diabetes Association
ATTN: National Call Center
1701 North Beauregard Street
Alexandria, VA 22311
Phone: 1–800–342–2383
Email: askADA@diabetes.org
Internet: www.diabetes.org/main/type1/complications/
    kidney/transplant.jsp

Medicare Coverage of Kidney Dialysis and Kidney Transplant Services
Publication Number CMS–10128
U.S. Department of Health and Human Services
Centers for Medicare & Medicaid Services
7500 Security Boulevard
Baltimore, MD 21244–1850
Phone: 1–800–MEDICARE (1–800–633–4227)
TDD: 1–877–486–2048
Internet: www.medicare.gov/publications/pubs/pdf/
    esrdcoverage.pdf

What Every Patient Needs To Know, 2004
United Network for Organ Sharing
P.O. Box 2484
Richmond, VA 23218
Phone: 1–888–TX–INFO–1 (894–6361)
Internet: www.unos.org

Newsletters and Magazines

Family Focus Newsletter (published quarterly)
National Kidney Foundation Inc.
30 East 33rd Street
New York, NY 10016
Phone: 1–800–622–9010
Email: info@kidney.org
Internet: www.kidney.org

For Patients Only (published six times a year)
ATTN: Subscription Department
18 East 41st Street
20th Floor
New York, NY 10017–6222

Renalife (published quarterly)
American Association of Kidney Patients
3505 East Frontage Road
Suite 315
Tampa, FL 33607
Phone: 1–800–749–2257
Fax: 813–636–8122
Email: info@aakp.org
Internet: www.aakp.org

Acknowledgments

The National Institute of Diabetes and Digestive and Kidney Diseases thanks these dedicated health professionals for their careful review of this publication.

Donald E. Hricik, M.D.
University Hospitals of Cleveland

Christopher Y. Lu, M.D.
University of Texas Southwestern Medical Center

The individuals listed here facilitated field testing for this publication. The NIDDK thanks them for their contribution.

Kim Bayer, M.A., R.D., L.D.
BMA Dialysis
Bethesda, MD

Cora Benedicto, R.N.
Clinic Director
Gambro Health Care
N Street Clinic
Washington, DC

About the Kidney Failure Series

You and your doctor will work together to choose a treatment that's best for you. The booklets and fact sheets of the NIDDK Kidney Failure Series can help inform you about the specific issues you will face.

Booklets

- *Kidney Failure: Choosing a Treatment That's Right for You*
- *Treatment Methods for Kidney Failure: Hemodialysis*
- *Treatment Methods for Kidney Failure: Peritoneal Dialysis*
- *Treatment Methods for Kidney Failure: Transplantation*
- *Eat Right to Feel Right on Hemodialysis*
- *Kidney Failure Glossary*

Fact Sheets

- *Kidney Failure: What to Expect*
- *Vascular Access for Hemodialysis*
- *Hemodialysis Dose and Adequacy*
- *Peritoneal Dialysis Dose and Adequacy*
- *Amyloidosis and Kidney Disease*
- *Anemia in Kidney Disease and Dialysis*
- *Renal Osteodystrophy*
- *Financial Help for Treatment of Kidney Failure*

Learning as much as you can about your treatment will help make you an important member of your health care team.

The NIDDK will develop additional materials for this series as needed. Please address any comments about this series and requests for copies to the National Kidney and Urologic Diseases Information Clearinghouse. Descriptions of the publications in this series are available at *www.kidney.niddk. nih.gov/kudiseases/pubs/kidneyfailure/index.htm.*

National Kidney and Urologic Diseases Information Clearinghouse

3 Information Way
Bethesda, MD 20892–3580
Phone: 1–800–891–5390
Fax: 703–738–4929
Email: nkudic@info.niddk.nih.gov
Internet: www.kidney.niddk.nih.gov

The National Kidney and Urologic Diseases Information Clearinghouse (NKUDIC) is a service of the National Institute of Diabetes and Digestive and Kidney Diseases (NIDDK). The NIDDK is part of the National Institutes of Health under the U.S. Department of Health and Human Services. Established in 1987, the Clearinghouse provides information about diseases of the kidneys and urologic system to people with kidney and urologic disorders and to their families, health care professionals, and the public. The NKUDIC answers inquiries, develops and distributes publications, and works closely with professional and patient organizations and Government agencies to coordinate resources about kidney and urologic diseases.

Publications produced by the Clearinghouse are carefully reviewed by both NIDDK scientists and outside experts.

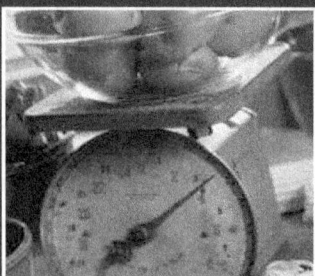

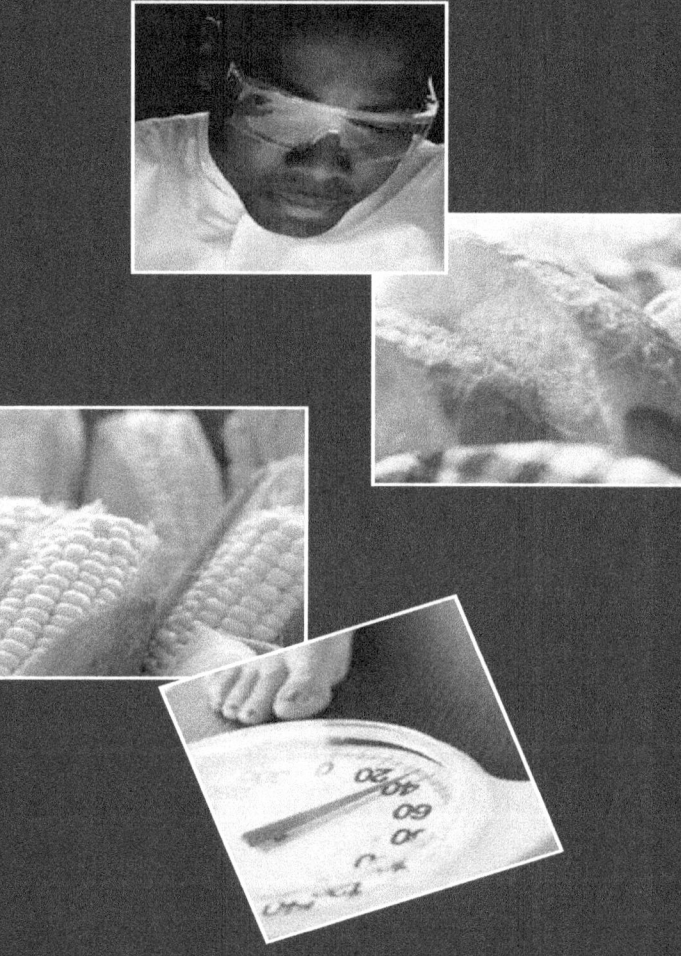

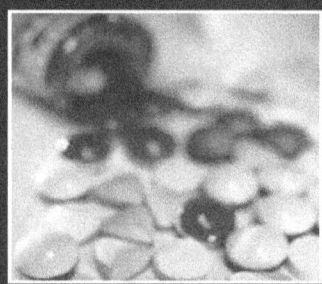

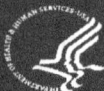 U.S. Department of Health and Human Services
National Institutes of Health

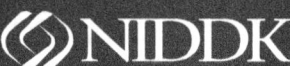NIDDK

National Institute of Diabetes and Digestive and Kidney Diseases
NIH Publication No. 06 4687
May 2006